W9-AVR-750

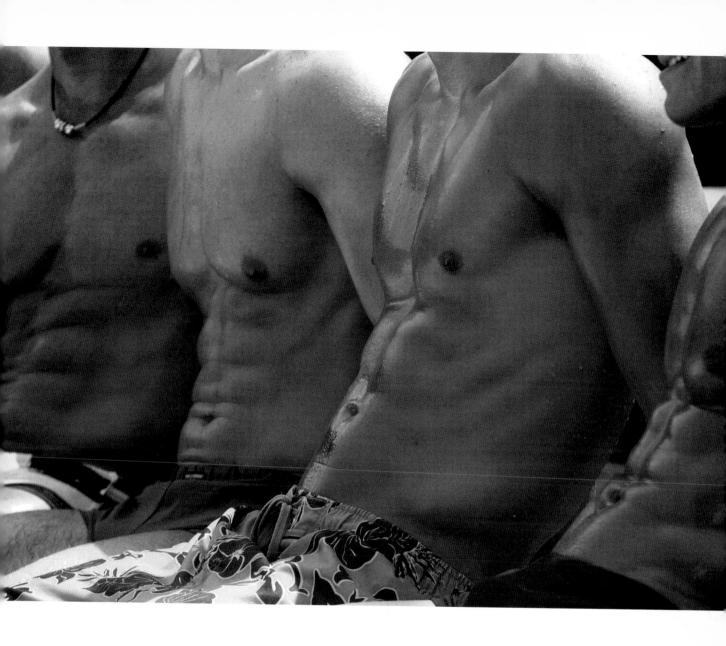

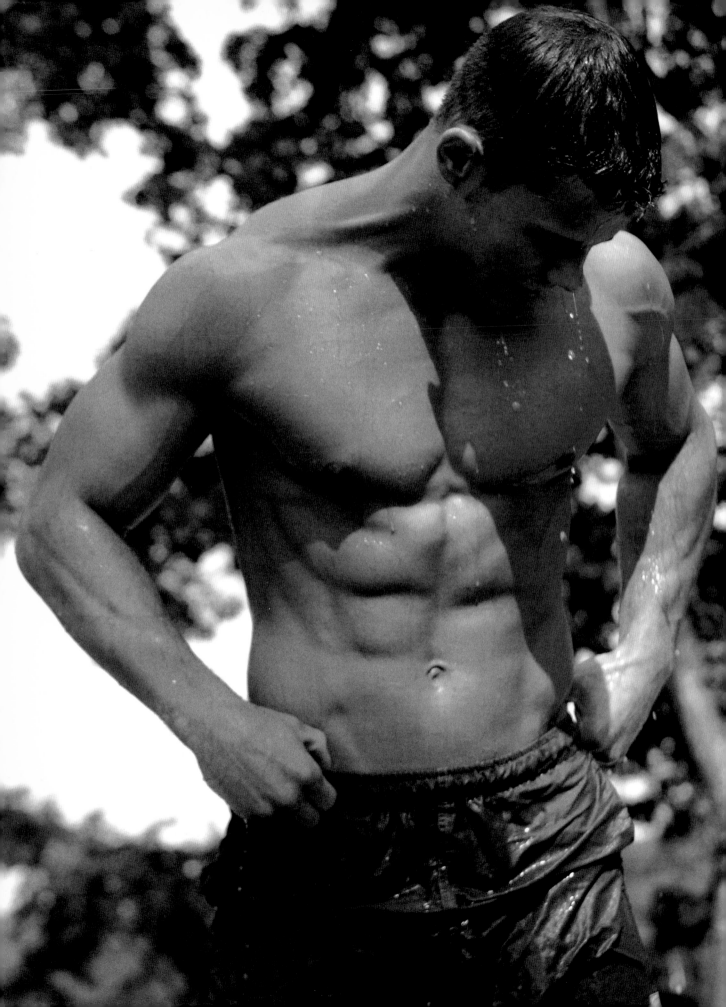

BEYOND BASIC TRAINING

FITNESS STRATEGIES FOR MEN

JON GISWOLD

PHOTOGRAPHS BY **AUGUSTUS BUTERA**

ST. MARTIN'S PRESS ≋ NEW YORK

ALSO BY JON GISWOLD

Basic Training: A Fundamental Guide to Fitness for Men

A Note to Readers: This book is for informational purposes only. Readers are advised to consult a doctor before beginning any exercise program.

www.stmartins.com

Designed and composed by Gretchen Achilles

Library of Congress Cataloging-in-Publication Data

Giswold, Jon.

Beyond basic training / Jon Giswold ; photographs by Augustus Butera.—1st U.S. ed.

p. cm.

ISBN 0-312-30755-1

1. Exercise for men. 2. Physical fitness for men. I. Title.

GV482.5.G58

613.7'1'081—dc21   2003046873

First Edition: November 2003

10 9 8 7 6 5 4 3 2 1

I heard something one day by chance that hit me with an impact so profound that it seemed perfect for the beginning of this acknowledgment page of my book—Information, without a system, is chaos. This book would be chaos without the passionate enthusiasm and vision of Elizabeth Beier. She trusted me enough to assemble this book my way, and I want to thank her for the giving me the system to make it work. Michael Connor for looking after Elizabeth, and to Michael Denneny for believing in me from the start.

This project would not look the way it does without the incredible talent of Augustus Butera. He and his unbelievable staff—Vanessa Rogers, Loraine Pantic, Dan Engel, and James Warren—went beyond my expectations in achieving the images for this book. The learning curve was steep, but the landing was smooth.

A special thanks goes out to Mike Lyons of the The Lyons Group (www.lyonsgroupny.com) for his continual support. The Lyons Group provided this project with models who are not only handsome and talented but are also sincere and good-hearted. Mike has that Midas touch when it comes to recognizing fresh talent and creates limitless opportunity for the following men: Adam Scorgie, Louis Gross, Jeff Herbert, Gregory Butler, Tyler Appleby, Andrew Aponick, Ted Trullinger, Matthew Foster-Moore, Peter Gaeth, Jordan Kitchen, Lawrence Bullock, Ivan Villegas, and Nico Nelson.

Personal friends who found their way onto the page for being superb athletes and role models include: John Ferris, Savvas Giautsis, Joe Petcka, Dean Dufford, Steve Jordan, David Kang, and Adam Figueroa.

Marc Wolinsky and Barry Skovgaard for the use of their breathtaking home in Water Mill, New York, and for being my best fans. Thank you to Larry Baker for feeding the guys and taking care of us all.

Ray Murray and Geert Maartens for the use of their home in Mattituck, New York, and for Ray's artful eye.

The men and women who are more than training clients, but my friends. They inspire me each and every session: Dan and Esty Brodsky, Jonathan Brodsky, Eileen Goudge and Sandy Kenyon, Jon and Joy Santlofer, Al and Claire Zuckerman, Ed McCabe, Lynn Pell, Candice Pell, Lauren Chiamotti, Larry Luckinbill, and Lucie Arnaz. I must thank all the men and women who continue to take classes with me around the world. As the saying goes, without you I am nothing.

Special thanks go out to Giovanni Falconi and Ana Vega for making my life easier, and Enid Stubin for my voice and her steady reassurance. I am grateful every day for the day I met my literary agent and good friend Ken Roberts.

Above all else, thank you Marc Raboy for staying beside me all these years. This is for Fanny.

GOING TO THE NEXT LEVEL

What do men need? George Carlin once joked that all self-help books are bogus (of course he used a different word), that getting to the store to buy a self-help book or motivational book proved that you were motivated simply by walking to the bookstore. You're motivated enough already! Turn around and go home! There is some truth to that. By picking yourself up and looking at this book, you have proved your motivation.

What men need and what men want are two separate things. I think men need options, direction—in other words, programming. Men are typically creatures of habit; once they find something that works or fits into their lives, they stick with it. Are you one of these men? I know I am. And it is important to consider. Look directly down the barrel of fear. Our fear of something new is fear of the unknown and/or the prediction of failure. Men do not like to fail. But we need to experiment and fail in order to change. In the many letters and e-mails I have received, men constantly ask about the desire to change. "How do I get my abs leaner?" "I'd like to put on some muscle, but I've been skinny my whole life. What should I do?" and "I'd like to build up to look like the guys in your book, but I don't belong to a gym. Can I still reach that goal?" These questions are honest indications that men want to change, but they don't know how. So they stick with the same routine: the same lunch, the same partner, and the same choices. *Beyond Basic Training* is a book that will offer you options. Most misconceptions and predetermined ideas of who should be doing yoga or ball training are just that. The truth is, these techniques are for every one. It is not my goal to have you fail. I want more than anything for you to succeed. I want you to change or at least to change your attitude about alternative practices. Do not turn away! You are going to find the benefits amazing. Let me get into your head and you'll find out why.

Beyond Basic Training will take you to a new level. With the current attention on Eastern disciplines and the resurrection of some tried-and-true techniques, the exercise landscape is not only becoming more and more confusing, it could cost a week's salary to buy a book for each practice and two weeks' vacation time to try them all! *Beyond Basic Training* synthesizes all of the trends of the new century and reintroduces the reader to some of the time-tested classics.

This book is broken up into three sections. Each section is comprised of information that will help you create a better body and better sense of your possibilities.

The first section, "Strategy," will help you better understand general fitness guidelines and formulas that will give you an edge when establishing a new workout routine. A client recently suggested to me that he was completely different from anyone else, and that his behavior and stubbornness in resisting exercise was unique to him. I hated to burst his bubble, but I had to make him aware that we are all very similar to each other. Our behavior keeps us from finding success. In this section you will find some exercises that will point out who you are and what keeps you from the gold medal, the spiritual calm, the success in creating the body you desire, and the self-esteem that goes along with that reachable goal.

Each strategy offers an introductory session of exercises for foundation building, a minimalist routine for time efficiency, and intermediate-level modifications of the same exercises to advance the intensity and create impressive results. This will guarantee a wide assortment of exercises to choose from so you can find the mix of training techniques that will be most effective for you.

In the "Getting Physical: Performance" section, you'll find strategies to enhance your current regimen or help you start an exercise routine. The chapter will explain where each strategy—say, Pilates—comes from. You'll learn if tools are needed in order to practice this strategy at home (balls, mats, etc.), and you'll be given a list of what to expect. Finally, the reader will be shown, through photographs and text, how to perform each exercise in each fitness strategy.

The third section, "Integration," will help you implement new attitudes about crosstraining and the benefits of heart-rate monitoring, nutritional strategies, stress management, and how to concentrate on overall better health.

Beyond Basic Training will help you break out of the dull, familiar routine you may now find yourself in and get you excited about the many options available. Crosstraining can change your fitness profile fast, and this new direction can be your guide.

A friend of mine asked me point-blank, "What is different about this book? DO we really need to read about how to do another bicep curl?" With a sea of fitness books and videotapes on the shelf, I knew what he meant. But I sold him on the concept of stability training and why it is important. He listened and agreed that the concept of balance training is vital to improve a person's fitness level and to inspire a new and improved training technique. But more importantly, he understood the need for a clear and attainable program choice. I think that people should have the choice to exercise at home and get the results that people in the health club world are offered. *Beyond Basic Training* is perfect for someone who wants dramatic results, but has limited time, funds, and resources. This book offers you a new and refreshing way to train.

Beyond Basic Training is about balance. If I can use one word to characterize this book it would be *balance*. It's what we strive for in every aspect of our lives. The balance between right and left, right and wrong, balancing our checkbook, overwork and underachievement, our personal relationships, and even our personal behavior lie in a delicate balance.

One of the first things we learn as infants is the ability to stand. Standing on two legs separates us from the animal kingdom. Standing requires balancing! Ask anyone who has an injury or weakness due to a disorder. In order to stand upright, you have to recruit muscle from your upper body, your lower body, and your midsection. Balance equals strength. By conditioning muscle systems, you can maintain balance and live a healthy, carefree life. Sounds too easy? It is easy. As we age, we lose balance. Studies have shown that after around the ages of twenty to twenty-five, our bodies begin to deteriorate. We cannot halt this part of the aging process, but we can modify it. Adding balance to physical training helps the body perform better. That's what all the buzz is about. You may have heard it called "functional training" or "natural strength." You can build a stronger body, create a stronger machine, and keep the aging process at bay by taking good care of yourself and modifying how you train.

Gravity keeps us all on Earth, right? Just because gravity is invisible doesn't mean that it doesn't have a resistance value. It places pressure on our spines as we stand and sit. The strength of our body systems keeps us upright. A major reason to consider taking up the type of strength training this book will introduce you to is to fight the effects of gravity. As with many "trends" in fitness, this philosophy isn't an overnight sensation. Many of the techniques in the following pages have been around for years, utilized by those on the search for better training models and by elite atheletes who have long used these methods to keep in ideal condition for their sport.

My goal is to get you to train for better life *function*. Function is integrated, multiplanar movement that involves acceleration, deceleration, and stabilization. In layman's terms, to function is to start, stop, and turn. Most strength and conditioning programs involve uniplanar (**sagittal plane**) force production, better known as pushing and pulling. Very little time is dedicated to neuromuscular stabilization training, core stabilization training, and **eccentric training** in all three planes of motion (*sagittal:* forward and back; *frontal:* side to side; and *transverse:* around).

A majority of exercisers perform strength-training programs on machines that have been designed without an understanding of functional anatomy, functional biomechanics, and human movement science. Machines provide artificial stabilization and only allow isolated, uniplanar training. This form of training is effective for **hypertrophy** (building muscle) but it does very little to improve daily function or prevent injury. Several machines have recently emerged and classic cable-system machines and resistance tubing, used for many years, have been reinvented to help solve this problem.

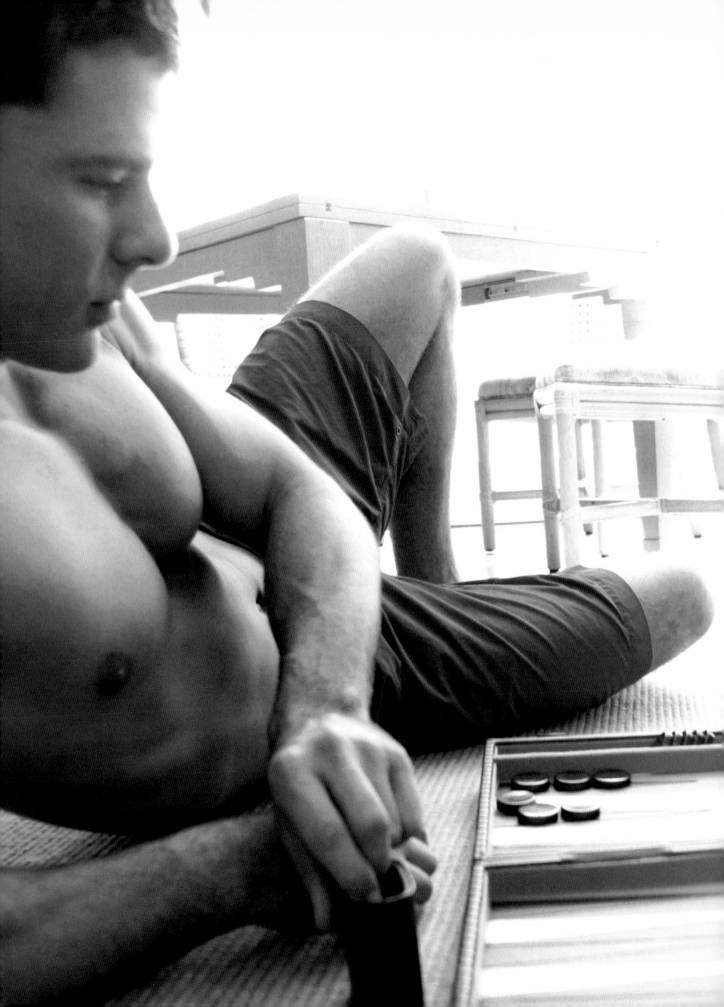

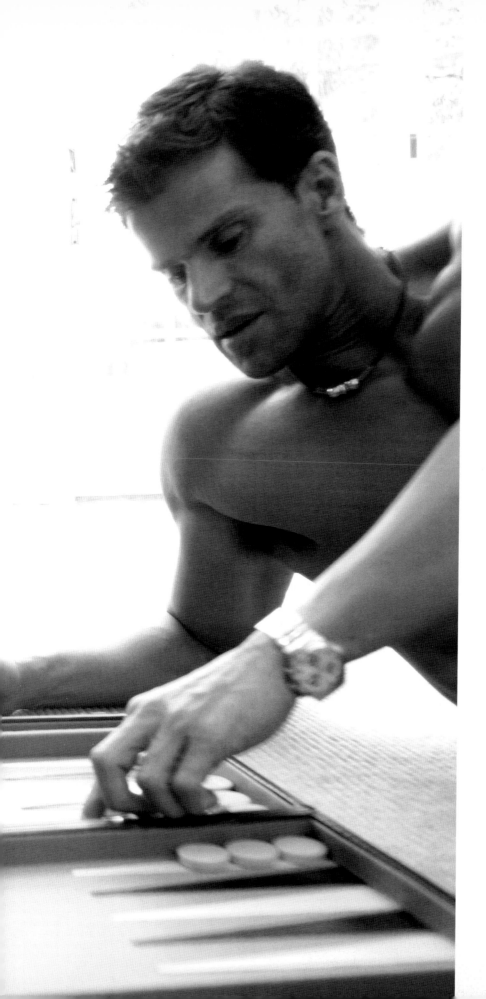

PART I

STRATEGY

(A carefully devised plan of action to achieve a goal/the art of developing or carrying out such a plan)

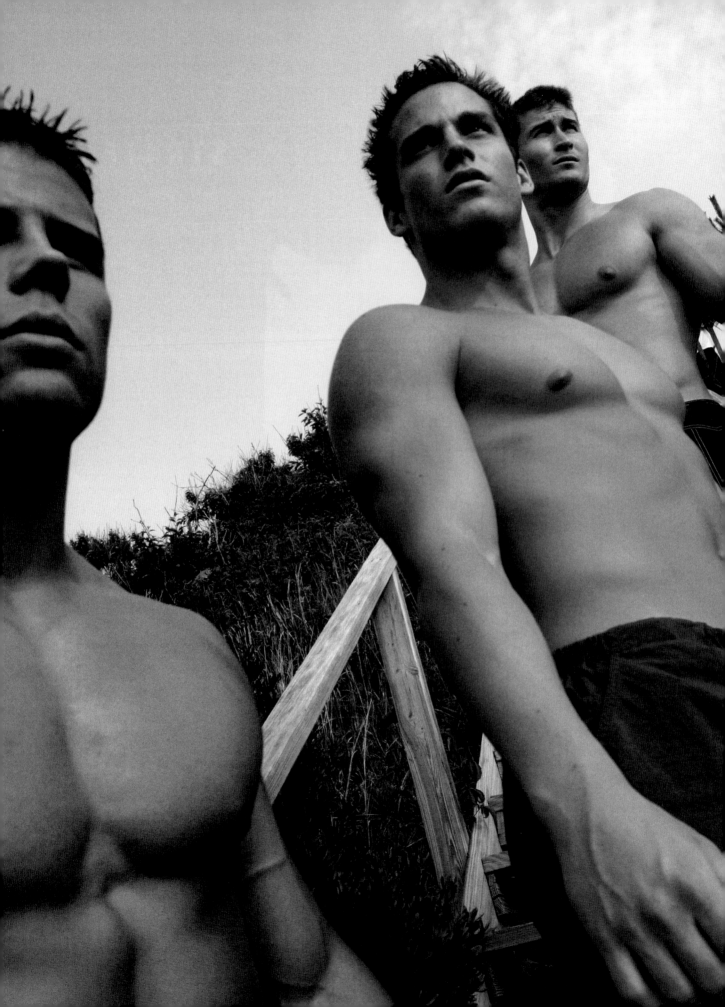

CHAPTER ONE

STRATEGY: TOOLS FOR WINNING

YOUR ROLE

Keep an open mind and allow yourself to explore the strategies introduced in this chapter. You picked up this book to look for direction. You want to be inspired. You want to see changes in your body and in your attitude. TRY.

MY ROLE

Let me be your coach. When you think of a coach who has influenced a great team or an inspirational leader, who do you think of? Why did you choose that person? What attributes does that person possess that urge people to follow him or her? I would like to be that person for you. I want you to learn something new and to find out not only how to perform exercises but how to feel better about yourself as a person. My job is to help people reach higher goals for themselves physically and emotionally.

As your coach, I want to try and bring you to a newfound appreciation of not only your body and physical ability, but of yourself as a person. My goal is to focus on *your* goals and help guide you to success by helping you understand yourself better and to identify some of the obstacles that could impede your success. I want you to find what you are looking for. That may sound simple, but the process can be filled with personal obstacles that you may be unaware of. These obstacles will always derail you unless you change the way you react toward them.

The hardest part of attempting something new is overcoming the fear of trying. After you try anything once, all you have to do from that point on is refine the task or practice until you excel at it.

TEN ELEMENTS TO CLARIFY YOUR FITNESS TRAINING PLAN.

1. What do you want from a fit lifestyle?

2. Who are you right now? Describe yourself.

3. How do you want to train?

4. What are your obstacles?

5. How will you reach your goal?

6. What makes you think you can succeed?

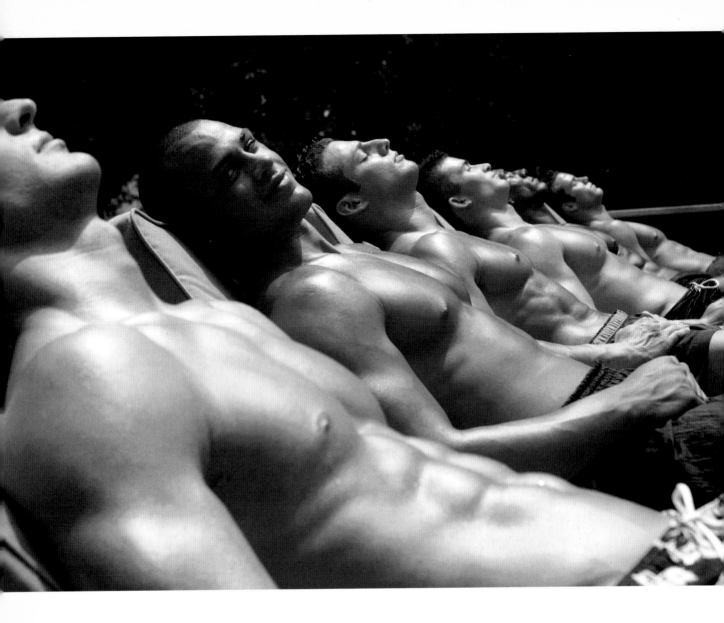

7. What technique will provide you with success?

8. What are your short-term goals?

9. What are your long-term goals?

10. Summary: What are the themes in each of the prior nine questions?

This is who you are!

CHAPTER TWO

GETTING TO KNOW YOU:
INVENTORY/SELF-EVALUATION

LIFE GAME: SELF-ESTEEM CHECKLIST

This game requires you to be honest in every true or false answer. If your answer would be "Sometimes," then answer "False" until you can honestly answer "True." If the question isn't applicable to you, then check "True."

There are fifteen questions in each category. Add up the total number of "True" checks in each section and record the figure. Add all the categories together to determine your total score.

Record your total and the date in a journal or your datebook. Compare your total to the total possible number of sixty points.

Play the game every six months until you achieve the goal of sixty points.

YOU AND YOUR ENVIRONMENT

	T	F
1. My home is clean and well kept.	☐	☐
2. I live in a house/apartment that I love.	☐	☐
3. I make my bed every day.	☐	☐
4. I recycle.	☐	☐
5. I have nothing in storage that I do not need.	☐	☐
6. My clothing is clean, pressed, and makes me look good.	☐	☐

YOU AND YOUR ENVIRONMENT (CONTINUED)

	T	F
7. My appliances and electrical equipment work perfectly.	☐	☐
8. My personal papers are neat and filed away.	☐	☐
9. My car works perfectly.	☐	☐
10. My sink is tidy and free of dirty dishes right now.	☐	☐
11. I have no unfinished home-repair projects.	☐	☐
12. I live in a city/town that I love.	☐	☐
13. My workstation is productive and inspiring.	☐	☐
14. My refrigerator is clean.	☐	☐
15. The food in my cupboard is fresh—not outdated.	☐	☐

MIND AND BODY

	T	F
1. I have a life beyond work.	☐	☐
2. I floss every day.	☐	☐
3. I have something to look forward to every day.	☐	☐
4. I do not use illegal drugs or misuse prescriptions.	☐	☐
5. My cholesterol is at a healthy level.	☐	☐
6. I have had a complete physical in the past two years.	☐	☐
7. I have no habits I find unacceptable.	☐	☐
8. I do not smoke.	☐	☐
9. My weight is within an ideal range.	☐	☐
10. I am taking care of my emotional or physical problems.	☐	☐
11. I exercise four to five times a week.	☐	☐
12. I have my eyes tested every two years.	☐	☐
13. I visit the dentist every year.	☐	☐

MIND AND BODY (CONTINUED)   T   F

14. I take care of my fingernails and toenails.   ☐   ☐

15. I limit my intake of alcohol.   ☐   ☐

OF THE HEART   T   F

1. I correspond with family and friends regularly.   ☐   ☐

2. I do not gossip about others.   ☐   ☐

3. I live my life on my own terms.   ☐   ☐

4. I do not judge or criticize others.   ☐   ☐

5. There is nothing unresolved with my past relationships.   ☐   ☐

6. I get along with my parents.   ☐   ☐

7. I get along with my siblings.   ☐   ☐

8. I have let go of relationships that were unhealthy for me.   ☐   ☐

9. I always tell the truth.   ☐   ☐

10. I quickly clear up miscommunications if needed.   ☐   ☐

11. I vote and participate in the democratic process.   ☐   ☐

12. I have a best friend.   ☐   ☐

13. There is no one I avoid.   ☐   ☐

14. I do not make self-deprecating statements.   ☐   ☐

15. I am reliable and stand by my word.   ☐   ☐

MONEY MONEY MONEY   T   F

1. I have no legal clouds hanging over me.   ☐   ☐

2. I currently live within my means.   ☐   ☐

3. I pay my bills on time.   ☐   ☐

	T	F
4. I have paid back money that I have borrowed.	☐	☐
5. I have insurance on all my assets.	☐	☐
6. I have medical insurance.	☐	☐
7. I have a financial plan in place for the future.	☐	☐
8. All of my tax returns have been paid.	☐	☐
9. I am paid well for my work.	☐	☐
10. My will is updated.	☐	☐
11. My checkbook is balanced.	☐	☐
12. I give to charitable causes once a year.	☐	☐
13. I know how much I am worth.	☐	☐
14. I have a nest egg to fall back on in case of emergency.	☐	☐
15. My career is one that I enjoy, and it enriches my life.	☐	☐

PERSONAL GROWTH ACTIONS

Take a risk—adventure

Learn a new language—personal growth

Find a spiritual outlet—soul

Try out a new hobby—creativity

Take a sexuality workshop—sensuality

Volunteer for a good cause—humanity

Go on a date with someone new or with your significant other—relationships

ANSWER THE FOLLOWING QUESTIONS AS THEY PERTAIN TO YOU NOW, OR AT ANY TIME IN THE PAST.

History of heart problems, chest pain, or stroke?   Yes ____   No ____

History of heart problems in immediate family?   Yes ____   No ____

Increased blood pressure?   Yes ____   No ____

Increased blood cholesterol?   Yes ____   No ____

Chronic illness or special condition?   Yes ____   No ____

Difficulty with physical exercise or activity?   Yes ____   No ____

Advice from a physician not to exercise?   Yes ____   No ____

Recent surgery (last twelve months)?   Yes ____   No ____

History of breathing or lung problems?   Yes ____   No ____

Cigarette smoking habit? Number per day?   ____

Obesity (as described by your physician)?   Yes ____   No ____

Diabetes or thyroid condition?   Yes ____   No ____

Hernia or any related condition?   Yes ____   No ____

Feelings of dizziness or loss of balance?   Yes ____   No ____

Immune system disorders
(sickness, allergies, etc . . .)?   Yes ____   No ____

Any orthopedic or muscular injuries?   Yes ____   No ____

Please provide a full and chronological account of your exercise history that begins with your involvement or noninvolvement in high school and college athletics. Cite any and all competitive, recreational, or seasonal sport activities that have followed in your adult years and include a brief history of the various exercise programs, fitness practices, and trainers you may have also incorporated up to the present time. Highlight your age for each activity, as well as its duration and frequency.

ACTIVITY:	AGE	DURATION	FREQUENCY

Do you have any negative feelings toward, or have you had any bad experiences with physical activity or exercise? Yes ___ No ___ (if yes, please explain)

_____

Briefly describe your current physical capacity in the following areas (i.e., strong and competitive or needs improvement):

CARDIOVASCULAR ENDURANCE:

_____

STRENGTH:

_____

_____

FLEXIBILITY:

_____

_____

SPORT SKILLS:

_____

_____

What words best describe how you view your body and its ability to perform? Why?

_____

Please list five specific things you would like to accomplish through exercise, regardless of how realistic you may be about your capacity to do so (i.e., run a five kilometer or triathlon, achieve weight loss/muscle gain, improve performance in golf or other sport, etc.).

1. _____

2. _____

3. _____

4. _____

5. _____

STRESS:

Stress takes on many forms that can be either positive or negative. Please list the predominant stress factors in your life, as they pertain to positive and negative factors.

POSITIVE STRESS FACTORS:

_____

_____

_____

_____

NEGATIVE STRESS FACTORS:

_____

_____

_____

_____

Please identify three things you do to relieve the unmanageable stress in your life?

1. _____

2. _____

3. _____

SLEEP PATTERNS:

How many hours of sleep do you get per night? _____

Do you typically fall asleep easily? _____

What is generally the last thing you do before bedtime? _____

Do you sleep lightly or soundly? _____

How would you describe the way you feel when you wake? _____

Briefly describe your general energy level and the moods you may experience during the course of the day, citing all noticeable changes:

Morning: _____
_____

Afternoon: _____
_____

Evening: _____
_____

In the fifteen years that I have been training and teaching group exercise, I have heard many stories that have inspired me to continue on this career path. Every person comes to fitness with a history or the motive to change his or her life. Often an event forces someone to look at changing their behavior—maybe a life-threatening disease or an accident, or a sudden awareness that the scale has crept up thirty pounds since college. These realizations can be wake-up calls.

Many people look at me and the rest of the fitness community as if they were looking into a fish bowl. All of the well-groomed and carefully accessorized men who hit the gym, not to mention the growing population of personal trainers, once started where you are right now.

In 1987, I had lived in New York City for six years pursuing my version of the "making it in New York" dream. Before getting involved in fitness, I was in the fashion industry. I had been a clothing salesman since I was thirteen years old in my small hometown in northern Wisconsin and had worked my way from the Twin Cities to the Big Apple. I landed a great job at Barneys New York and, with the contacts I made, went to work selling menswear for Alexander Julian in his New York showroom. That experience led me to the idea that I could open my own design business and sell my own line of menswear. I had been designing for a few private clients and set my sights on a giant goal. This is also the time I met and started a relationship with my partner Marc. That period also introduced me to a fast-lane life of celebrities and nightlife. Small-town boy makes it in a high-profile industry in the Big City. But all of that came with a price: namely drugs and alcohol.

Then one night I discovered cocaine. It didn't take me long to become a daily user. The trouble was, I could function fairly well, or at least I thought I could. With my ego fed by a daily dose of coke and a desire to succeed in the highly competitive world of retail fashion, my addiction escalated. Isolation from most of my friends, having no nine-to-five schedule to keep, allowed me to snort more coke than work and the paranoia that comes along with that drug use set the stage for the next chain of events.

I had been on a three-day coke binge, drinking six-pack after six-pack of beer to dilute the edge of my anxiety, when I found myself sitting on the ledge of the window, on the eighth floor of the building we were living in on Nineteenth Street in Chelsea. It was the middle of the night. No sounds reached me other than the occasional cab whisking down Seventh Avenue or a distant horn. It seemed as though there was no way off that ledge other than plummeting down to the street. It seemed the right thing to do. It seemed like the *only* thing to do. But I remember having to pee. I thought that I would get up and go and pee and then jump. This is truly what was going through my mind. I didn't know how else I could stop my heart from beating so fast and my mind from spinning hopeless thoughts of inadequacy and negativity. On the outside I was the ever-optimistic Jon, but on the inside I was a drug addict—nothing more.

I climbed off the ledge to go into the bathroom and I caught a glimpse of myself in the mirror behind the dining table. I weighed less than 150 pounds, and in my underwear I looked like a concentration camp prisoner. My eyes were sunken into my forehead, dried blood crusted my nostrils from the two grams of cocaine I had consumed over the last few days. My skin was gray, and my spirit broken. I froze at the sight of myself in the mirror, and it was as if a light switched on in my soul. I cried. I thought that I had already died and this was my punishment—nonexistence. I had no feelings and no appetite to live. But in that moment I *saw* myself. I cried harder. I cried for the man I had become and for the power I had given up to drugs and booze. I cried so hard it hurt.

But hurting meant that I was still alive, alive in a way that I had not been in several months. This was my threshold. I walked through it knowing that I would have to make a dramatic change in my life in order to live. I fell asleep on the floor after writing a pledge to Marc and to myself for a new life.

The next day I went to an AA meeting. I hoped that I would find answers and people who could help me, but I was scared and alone in my own head. The room was filled with kind faces with eyes that could see directly into my bruised spirit. I sat there as quietly as I could, listening to the words and stories that seemed to make sense but that seemed so foreign at the same time. I knew it was important at least to speak my name and begin the process. I raised my hand. "Hi, my name is Jon. I am a drug addict and an alcoholic."

The next day I found myself on what they call a pink cloud. Feeling as if I had taken a giant step forward, I went to work, only to find that the space I was sharing was no longer a space I was welcome in. My papers had been packed up alongside a few boxes of sweaters and pants, sitting next to the door. I was told to find a new place to run my business. My first feeling was shame and then anger. How could this be happening when I was trying to get everything together? But it *was* happening, and the only thing I could do was grab my stuff and go.

With my boxes in tow, I went looking for a space to set up my floundering business. Somehow I trusted each step I was taking. I found a sign that said OFFICE FOR RENT on Twenty-second Street, just off Sixth Avenue, in the warehouse section of the Flatiron District (one block away from my publishing house). The office was a three-hundred-square-foot space adjacent to a printing business. I knew this office would be mine. In such a fragile state, I wasn't sure the landlord would want me as a tenant. His name was Ray, and he was a nice guy. For $350 a month, I could move in that day.

I was going to get the rest of my things and was waiting for the traffic light on Sixth Avenue to change when I heard a female voice say, "Is your name Jon?" I didn't respond. A tap on my shoulder. "Excuse me, are you Jon?" I nodded. "I heard you speak at a meeting the other night, and I was wondering how you're doing." I looked at an open face and inviting eyes and felt as though I mattered. The simplest of gestures can make a world of difference. I felt I had joined the human race again, like I had a place in it. The woman invited me to her exercise studio, which just happened to be across the street from my new office space. I agreed and stepped directly into a change that would dramatically affect my life and career. I stepped into my future.

Molly Fox Studios became a home away from home, an educational institution, a safe house and temple for many others and me. I was introduced to group exercise, which was just beginning to find its popularity in the United States. Jane Fonda was the toast of the industry, and Molly and her team of teachers were inventing new exercise methods and creating new techniques. I wanted in on this not-so-well-kept secret. My business had all but dried up. The stock market collapse of October 1987 essentially ended my design business, and I immersed myself in exercise. I took low-impact classes, body-sculpting classes, high/lo-impact, funk dance, abs classes, and stretch and tone. I could not get enough. Sometimes I took two or three classes a day. When I wasn't in class, I attended meetings. I was getting better. I was getting stronger. I was finding Jon.

I looked upon the men and women who taught Molly Fox's classes as idols. They radiated health and well-being. I knew that I wanted this to be my life. It was as if someone had tailor-made this career for me. Teaching offered everything that I wanted. It required expression, dance and movement, physical rushes and concrete results, applause, and a connection with people. There was no money in the field unless you earned it. We were paid twenty dollars an hour and one dollar a head over ten people. Today, that seems like nothing, but the first class I taught, where I had three people in my class, still remains one of the highlights of my life. I worked hard at fine-tuning my class and creating choreography, getting myself certified by fitness associations, and becoming an educator. Molly had high standards and expected the same of her staff. I was on my way. At the same time that I was finding my professional self, I was finding my *true* self. This time in my life gave me back my life. I am grateful each and every day that I work in the exercise field and can inspire others to get fit.

Molly Fox will always be my mentor and hero. I truly owe her more than thanks. She and I counted our first ninety days of sobriety together, and she invited me into a world that would have passed me by had she not tapped me on the shoulder and exercised the simplest form of humanity, an act of kindness.

GET OVER IT AND ON WITH IT

There comes a time when you have to take charge of your mind, your body, and your behavior. Whatever pushed the buttons that caused you to be defeated needs to be replaced. It's time to trade in your history for the present.

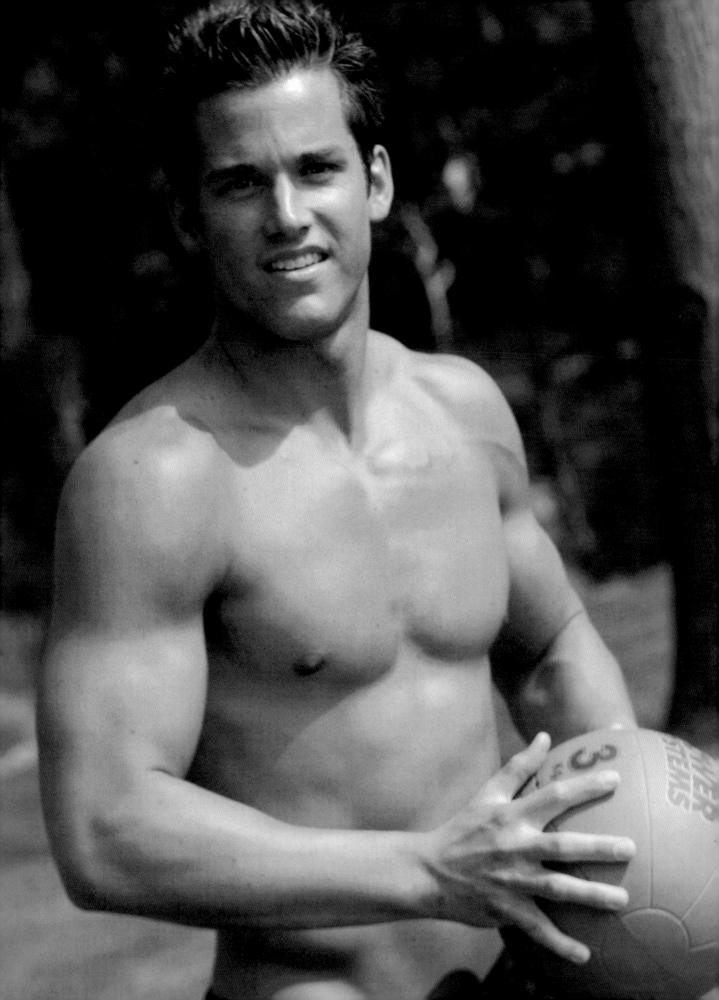

READY, SET . . . BEFORE YOU GO

Before you begin to exercise, consult with a qualified health practitioner, such as your physician. A preexercise assessment will help you determine the safest, most appropriate way to start your program.

Next, determine your short-term and long-term goals. Pursuing attainable goals will increase your self-esteem and self-confidence. Don't worry if you're feeling nervous about beginning an exercise program. Everybody does!

THE BIG THREE PLUS ONE

Your exercise program should concentrate on the following areas:

IMPROVING AEROBIC ENDURANCE.
For aerobic exercise, your choices are numerous. Swimming and water exercise are excellent because they don't place a lot of stress on the joints. Stationary and seated

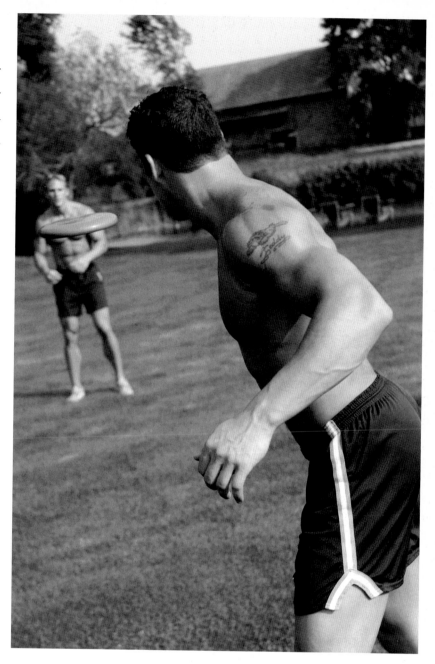

(known as recumbent) cycling are less stressful on the back and legs than some activities, and fitness walking is also a good option.

Try to follow the guidelines from the Centers for Disease Control and Prevention (CDC) and the American College of Sports Medicine (ACSM). These guidelines recommend that you accumulate forty minutes or more of moderate-intensity physical activity four or more days of the week.

INCREASING STRENGTH. Resistance training has gained considerable popularity with older adults over the last decade. It has been shown to stimulate bone growth, improve posture, decrease the percent of body fat, and improve balance and mobility. To ensure you train properly and effectively, procure the expertise of a certified personal trainer or instructor and have him or her design an appropriate resistance exercise program for you. (In fact, seeking the support of one of these professionals can help you adhere to the correct exercise safety guidelines and maximize the effectiveness of all types of exercise.)

IMPROVING FLEXIBILITY. You need to perform flexibility exercises in a slow, sustained manner, holding the stretches for up to thirty seconds. Make sure you feel the stretch in the muscles, rather than the joints. It is okay to stretch daily. Stretches for the backs of the legs, fronts of the legs, low back, and shoulders are recommended. These flexibility stretches are best performed at the end of the workout.

CORE TRAINING. The plus in our list. Core training has gained popularity, not because of the endless six-packs that grace the pages of every magazine or the rack of abs that every soap star displays, but because "core" has become the latest trend in the fitness industry. It stabilizes the low back and pelvis and works to maintain proper posture and body alignment as we move through our daily activities. Once the core has been established, there are few changes that need to be added to a regular fitness routine. The biggest change may be to start using your core to hold your body position and alignment while working out.

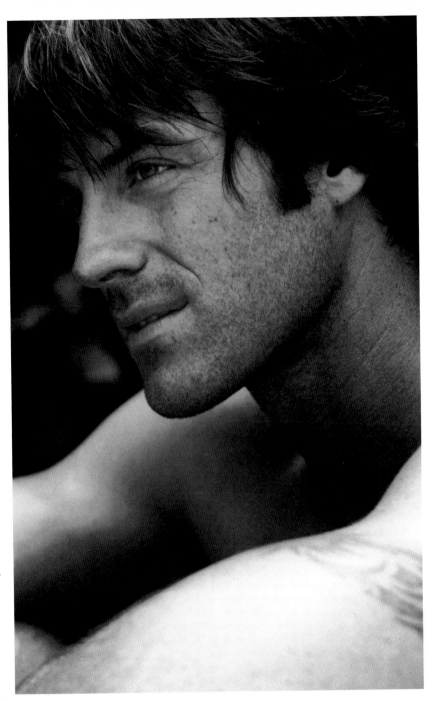

BEFORE YOU START AN EXERCISE PROGRAM, QUESTION YOURSELF

There are a few questions to ask yourself to determine whether you should see your doctor first.

Your first step is to ask yourself how active you want to be. This may sound like a silly question— you're probably planning on doing whatever you're capable of, whether that's a slow walk around the block or a vigorous step class. But if you're of a certain age or have certain cardiovascular risk factors, you may need to see your physician before beginning a program that involves vigorous (as opposed to moderate) aerobic activity.

HERE'S HOW EXERCISE INTENSITIES ARE TYPICALLY DEFINED

LOW-TO-MODERATE. This is an intensity that can be sustained relatively comfortably for a long period of time (about sixty minutes). This type of exercise typically begins slowly, progresses gradually, and usually isn't competitive in nature.

VIGOROUS. This is an intensity that is high enough to significantly raise both your heart and breathing rates and is usually performed for about twenty minutes before fatigue sets in.

Are you planning to participate in vigorous activities and are a man over forty? You should receive a medical exam first. The same is true for individuals of any age with two or more coronary artery disease risk factors (see page 24). If you're unsure if this applies to you, check with your physician.

MORE QUESTIONS

Now that you've made it through the first questions, there are a few more to answer. A "yes" to any ONE of the following questions means you should talk with your doctor, by phone or in person, BEFORE you start an exercise program. Explain which questions you answered "yes" to and the activities you are planning to pursue.

1. Have you been told you have a heart condition and should only participate in physical activity recommended by a doctor?

2. Do you feel pain (or discomfort) in your chest when you do physical activity? When you are not participating in physical activity? While at rest, do you frequently experience fast, irregular heartbeats or very slow beats?

3. Do you ever become dizzy and lose your balance, or lose consciousness? Have you fallen more than twice in the past year (no matter what the reason)?

4. Do you have a bone or joint problem that could worsen as a result of physical activity? Do you have pain in your legs or buttocks when you walk?

5. Do you take blood pressure or heart medications?

6. Do you have any cuts or wounds on your feet that don't seem to heal?

7. Have you experienced unexplained weight loss in the past six months?

8. Are you aware of any reason why you should not participate in physical activity?

If you answered no to all of these questions, you can be reasonably sure that you can safely take part in at least a moderate physical activity program. But again, if you are over forty and want to exercise more vigorously, you should check with your physician before getting started. By taking the time to evaluate whether you are ready to start exercising, you've planted yourself firmly on the path to better health and fitness.

CORONARY ARTERY DISEASE RISK FACTORS

Age (men over forty-five, women over fifty-five)

Family history of heart attack or sudden death

Current cigarette smoking

High blood pressure

High cholesterol

Diabetes

Physical inactivity

ACSM GUIDELINES FOR HEALTHY AEROBIC ACTIVITY

The American College of Sports Medicine (ACSM) recommends the following:

Exercise five times a week.

Warm up for five to ten minutes before aerobic activity.

Maintain your exercise intensity for thirty to forty-five minutes.*

Gradually decrease the intensity of your workout, then stretch to cool down during the last five to ten minutes.

FITTING IN FITNESS

One of the most popular excuses for failing to work out is not having enough time. Are you really so busy it is impossible to squeeze in exercise? Or is it more likely your time is spent on things that are not top priorities for you? If you frequently use lack of time as an excuse for missing workouts, fill in the following chart.

YOUR USE OF TIME

Being totally objective, fill out the following top-ten list with items that are most important to you, ranking them in order of importance. Think in terms of your overall life and what you love the most.

TOP TEN THINGS IN MY LIFE

1. _____
2. _____
3. _____
4. _____
5. _____
6. _____
7. _____
8. _____
9. _____
10. _____

Now list the top ten ways you currently spend your time, from the most to the least time consuming.

TOP TEN WAYS I USE MY TIME

1. _____
2. _____
3. _____
4. _____
5. _____

*If weight loss is your major goal, participate in your activity for at least forty minutes for five days each week.

6 _____

7. _____

8. _____

9. _____

10. _____

Take a look at list 2. From that list and your experience, note any activities that whittle away at least ten minutes of your time a day. Include things like waiting in store lines, waiting on hold on the phone, being stuck in traffic, waiting for clients, watching TV, etc. Beside each entry, state how much time gets spent and add up your average daily total.

TIME I WASTE DAILY

1. _____

2. _____

3. _____

4. _____

5. _____

6 _____

7. _____

8. _____

9. _____

10. _____

TOTAL WASTED TIME EACH DAY

(HOURS/MINUTES): _____

WAYS OF INCREASING TIME FOR FITNESS

Compare list 1 with list 2. Do you devote the majority of your time to what means the most to you? Or do you find yourself using precious time on activities that really don't mean that much? If your two lists do not enhance each other, it is time to get your priorities in line. For example, if your number-one priority is enjoying your family, yet you work long, hard days to support them, you may need to look at working shorter days for less pay.

Now look at list 3. The purpose of this exercise is twofold. First, it shows we all waste time. After all, no one can be expected to run full tilt without a moment of rest. There is always time available for health and fitness; it is simply a matter of motivation. (If you won the lottery, wouldn't you find time to pick up the money?) Second, this list shows that planning your time more wisely can free up other parts of the day. For example, if you find yourself holding on the telephone a lot, use that time to pay bills or make a grocery list. While you are waiting in a doctor's office or under a hair drier, why not catch up on your work-related reading? Then you will have effortlessly saved yourself a chunk of time for exercise and other fun things.

How much do you value yourself? If you pack the day so full there is no time for you, you are stressing yourself beyond human limits. The body and mind need exercise and rest to stay fit and well. Take a closer look at your use of time to find a way to ease activity into your lifestyle.

HOW DO YOU MEASURE UP? TESTING—ONE, TWO, THREE

It seems we are all trying to get into better shape and enhancing our lives by eating healthier, cutting out or back on vices, and getting regular exercise. But how are we doing? Sure, you can fly on that new elliptical machine they just put in at the gym, but can you climb several flights of stairs if the elevator in your building is out of service?

Ask yourself:

Can you walk at a fast pace for ten minutes without feelings out of breath? = AEROBIC FITNESS

Can you run the last couple of blocks to a meeting you're running late for without collapsing? = ANAEROBIC POWER

Can you lug a full briefcase and/or a backpack around without feeling totally exhausted? = UPPER BODY STRENGTH

Can you surf the Internet without sitting hunched over your computer? = CORE STRENGTH

Can you balance on one foot to tie your sneakers? = BALANCE

Can you pick up a coin without bending your knees? = FLEXIBILITY

Does the waistband of your pants stay flat (without folding over) when you go beltless? = BODY FAT

If the answer to any of these questions is **no**, you should find out how you measure up. The following tests will provide you with a foundation for setting up a program that will boost your performance in all real-life areas, not just at the gym. You may look great from all the work lifting and running, but can you improve your performance overall in the real world, a world where you have to run after buses, lift cartons to the top shelf in your closet, sit up during an important meeting, move easily through a spirited game of volleyball, or just enjoy a good night's sleep? You will benefit by training in all areas of fitness. The body beautiful is great to look at, but a strong and capable body is even more satisfying. Don't leave a weak link in the chain, especially if you are building and training the "show me" areas.

To take the following short tests you'll need a second hand on your watch or clock, a standard chair, and a measuring tape (Yikes!). The tests are graded for a man between the ages of twenty-seven to forty-one years of age. The results for a younger man would involve a lower heart-rate count and higher repetitions in the strength test. Remember that you are only testing yourself, and the results are for your information only. How you use what you find out is up to you as well.

AEROBIC WALK. Walk for ten minutes as quickly as you can without breaking into a jog. Then take your heart rate by touching your neck next to your Adam's apple with your fingertips for ten seconds. Multiply that count by six, which equals how many times your heart beats per minute of aerobic exercise. Results vary with different ages. A score of under 90 is excellent, 90–100 is good, 100–25 is fair, over 125 needs some work.

"HOME" WORK—Walk three times per week for at least thirty minutes at about 3.5 miles per hour.

ANAEROBIC CLIMB. Walk up about forty to fifty steps without stopping. If you need to go up and

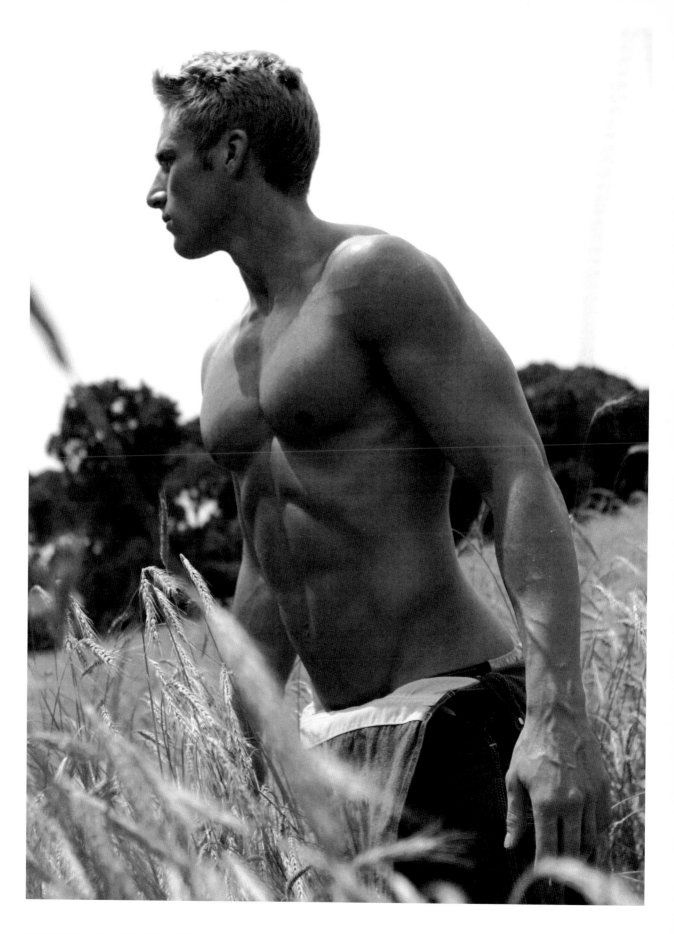

down a single flight of stairs then do so. Wait sixty seconds before you take your heart rate, as described above, on the neck for ten seconds (multiply by six). Under 90 is excellent, 90–100 is good, 100–25 is fair, and over 125 needs improvement.

> **"HOME" WORK**—Climb stairs in place of taking elevators.

UPPER BODY STRENGTH—PUSH-UPS. Hooray for the standard push-up! In the traditional push-up position, with both hands on the floor slightly wider than your shoulders and on your toes with your legs extended, count as many push-ups you can do without stopping or losing your technique. Over fifty is excellent, thirty-five to fifty is good, twenty to thirty-five is fair, and under twenty means you need to improve.

> **"HOME" WORK**—Try doing two sets of twelve to twenty push-ups every day.

CORE STRENGTH—CRUNCHES. Lie on the floor with your knees bent and your feet flat on the floor. With your hands behind your head, curl your upper body toward your lower body enough to clear your shoulder blades off the floor. Count as many crunches as you can before you feel you have to stop. Fifty-five and over is excellent, forty to fifty five is good, twenty-five to forty is fair, and under that needs improvement.

> **"HOME"WORK**—Try doing two sets of twenty-five to thirty crunches every day after your push-ups.

BALANCE—ONE-FOOT STAND. You may think that knowing how to balance is obvious, but balance requires both strength and concentration. As people age, they may lose their ability to balance. Stand on your strongest leg (the same side as the side you write) with your knee slightly bent. Raise the other leg, lifting your foot about two inches off the floor while keeping your arms relaxed at your side. Try to balance for at least thirty seconds. Over thirty seconds is excellent, twenty to thirty is good, eleven to twenty is fair, and if you can only manage fewer than ten, stay away from the balance beam.

> **"HOME" WORK**—Perform the one-foot stand holding the leg up for five seconds, ten times on each leg, three times a week.

FLEXIBILITY—TOE TOUCH. Stand with your feet separated a hip-width apart, with your knees slightly bent to unlock the joints. Bend forward from the hip joint, allowing your arms to reach toward the floor until you feel a comfortable stretch. Note how close your hands come to the floor. Slowly return to a standing position. Hands flat on the floor is excellent, touching the top of your shoes is good, touching your ankles is fair, and touching your midshin requires some attention.

> **"HOME" WORK**—Lie down on the floor with your knees bent. Lift one leg in the air with a towel or belt positioned over your toes. Extend the leg holding onto the belt/towel and gently pull on your foot until you feel a good stretch, holding for twenty to thirty seconds. Repeat with the other leg. Try doing this every day.

BODY FAT—AND THE ANGRY INCH

The cruelest test of them all. Strip. Take a look at yourself in the mirror, a good look. Trying pinching the skin away from muscle in three key areas: the chest, on the outer side between the nipple and the armpit; the waist, two inches from your belly button or the love handle area; the leg, on the inner side of the thigh. Use your index finger and thumb. If you cannot pinch any fat away from these areas, call me. If you can pinch an inch or more of fat away in any of these areas, the red flag has been raised.

> **"HOME" WORK**—Increase your cardio routine in duration or intensity and take an honest look at what you're eating.

Most health clubs and fitness centers with a staff of trainers can provide a methodical exam you can take to find out your exact measurements in a more scientific way. It is a good idea to have a formal assessment before you begin a workout routine to identify the areas that need work and to get an overall estimation of how fit you are. This test is a casual way for you to test your levels in the privacy of your own home. For those who pursue a regular fitness routine, it can also be a nice way to see progress and the results you have worked so hard for.

BATTLING BOREDOM

Do you find it difficult to get out of bed in the morning for your daily walk and easy to make up excuses to skip the gym on the way home? Even the most dedicated exercisers occasionally get bored with their routine. Waning motivation, cutting workouts short, and not feeling your old enthusiasm are all signs of a stale exercise regimen.

QUICK FIX

Evaluate your current routine to determine which part of it really bores you. A new variation on your favorite activity—such as cardiofunk or kickboxing instead of step aerobics, or hoisting free weights instead of working on machines—may be enough to reinvigorate a stale routine.

If you've always worked out indoors, logging miles on a treadmill, stairclimber, or stationary bike, move your workout outside for a change of scenery. Run, hike, or bike on trails; swim in a lake or ocean.

BIGGER CHANGES

When tweaking your routine isn't enough, make bigger changes. Take up an entirely new activity—especially something you never thought you'd do. If you've always stuck to solitary pursuits, sign up for a team sport, such as volleyball, basketball, or even doubles tennis. Or tackle something you've always shied away from—indulge your thirst for adventure with a rock-climbing class (start on an indoor wall, then move to the real thing as your skills improve).

GOOD COMPANY

Working out alone can provide an oasis of solitude in a busy day, but maybe you need some company. Exercise companions add a social element to any routine. Ask a friend to be your workout partner—you won't skip a workout if someone is waiting for you.

Just about every sport or activity has a club; to find one, ask around at gyms or local community centers. Keeping up with the crowd also means you'll be challenged to improve your skills. Ask about organized workouts and fun runs offered by local track clubs, as well as group rides hosted by cycling clubs. These

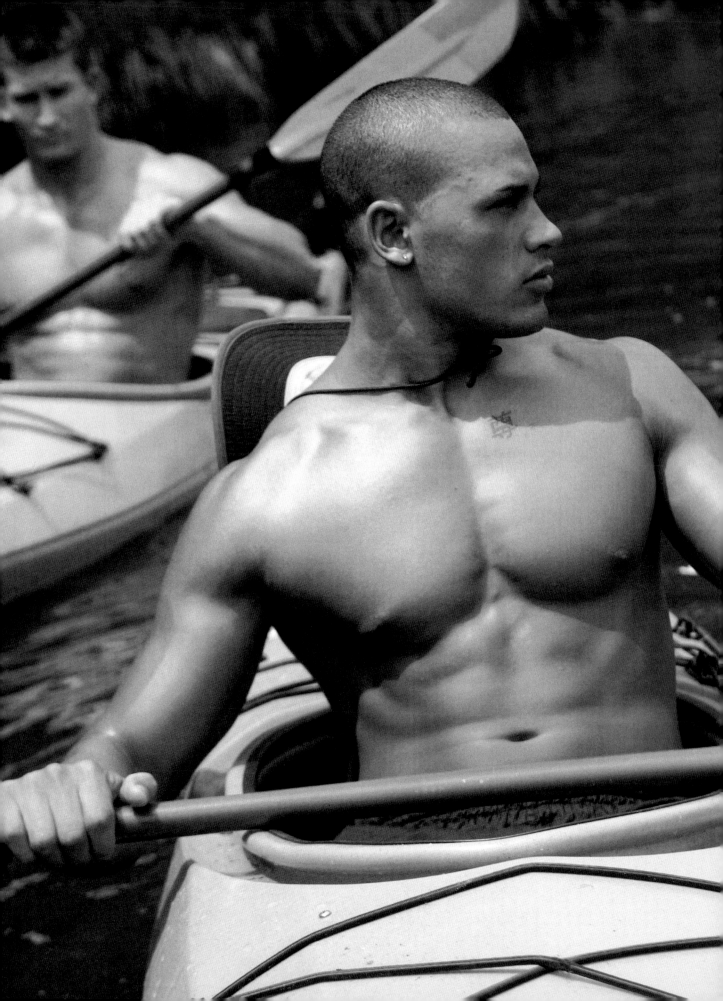

clubs also develop a community of others who share the same interest in a healthy lifestyle.

CHALLENGE YOURSELF

Many exercisers work out simply to stay in shape, and that's a worthy goal. But setting a big goal, such as finishing a ten-kilometer race or completing a rough-water swim, will give your daily workouts more meaning.

Start by incorporating bursts of speed into your workouts. After a gentle warm-up, alternate a fast pace with a slower one for recovery. This can be as simple as sprinting to the next tree or as structured as running intervals on a track or sprinting laps in the pool.

ADD VARIETY

Elite triathletes pioneered crosstraining, and it works for the rest of us, too. If you usually focus on one activity, substitute another a few days a week. Ideally, any exercise program includes elements of cardiovascular exercise, weight training, and flexibility.

NEW TOYS

Small exercise gadgets aren't necessary, but they can make your workouts more fun and challenging. Heart-rate monitors, aquatic toys, such as buoys and gloves, and safety equipment are just a few items to consider. Find out which new training gadgets are available for your favorite activity.

TAKE A BREAK

Sometimes you really do need time off. In that case, cut back on your usual routine and substitute other ac-

tivities. You might even find some that you enjoy more than your old favorites.

Once you've fought your first battle with boredom, you'll know the tricks to keep exercise from becoming too routine. Trying new sports, new classes, and new activities—and learning how to spice up old favorites—can help you overcome the inclination to devise creative excuses for not working out.

SLOWING THE AGING CLOCK

As you grow older, you may feel there is nothing you can do about the physiological changes that occur with aging. Surprise! There *is* something you can do, and it needn't even cost anything. What is it? *Exercise!*

THE AGE ANTIDOTE

Research has discovered the following in exercisers over the age of seventy.

- Physical activity in elders has been linked to the prevention of some cancers, as well as reduced risk of heart disease, hypertension, osteoporosis, obesity, Type 2 diabetes, and osteoarthritis.

- Mature adults who maintain high levels of cardiovascular endurance, strength, and flexibility are less likely to need long-term care.

- Falls, which are the leading cause of fatal injuries in people over seventy-five years old, can be reduced dramatically through participation in exercise programs that improve balance and mobility.

- Increased strength improves gait and bodily control and helps individuals function independently.

- Exercise is often associated with more effective stress

management, fewer sleep disorders, enlightened mental outlook, reduced loneliness, and lowered depression and anxiety.

Your training heart-rate zone is a critical element in exercise. Taking your pulse and figuring your heart rate during a workout is one of the primary ways to ascertain the intensity level at which you and your heart are working. There are many ways to measure exercise intensity. The Karvonen Formula is one of most effective methods used to determine heart rate. Rating Perceived Exertion (RPE) and talk-test methods are subjective measurements that can be used in addition to taking a pulse.

THE KARVONEN FORMULA

This is a heart-rate reserve formula and one of the most effective methods used to calculate training heart rate. The formula factors in your resting heart rate, so first, you'll need to determine your resting heart rate by doing the following:

- Prior to getting out of bed in the morning, take your pulse on your wrist (radial pulse) or on the side of your neck (carotid pulse).

- Count the number of beats, starting with zero, for one minute. If you don't have a stop watch or a clock with a second hand in your bedroom, you can measure the time by watching the number change on a digital alarm clock. Find your pulse and start counting when the minute number changes; stop counting when it changes again.

- To help assure accuracy, take your resting heart rate three mornings in a row and average the three numbers.

The next step in finding your training heart-rate zone is determining the intensity level at which you should exercise. As a general rule, you should exercise at an intensity between 50 to 85 percent of your heart-rate reserve. Your individual level of fitness will ultimately determine where you fall within this range. Use the following table as a guide for determining the best intensity level for you:

BEGINNER OR LOW-FITNESS LEVEL	50%-60%
AVERAGE FITNESS LEVEL	60%-70%
HIGH FITNESS LEVEL	75%-85%

Once you've determined and gathered this information, pull it together with the Karvonen Formula:

220 – AGE = MAXIMUM HEART RATE; THEN MAXIMUM HEART RATE – RESTING HEART RATE × INTENSITY + RESTING HEART RATE = TRAINING HEART RATE

For example, Eric is thirty-three years old, has a resting heart rate of seventy-five and he's just beginning his exercise program (his intensity level will be 50 to 60 percent). Eric's training heart-rate zone will be 131 to 142 beats per minute:

ERIC'S MINIMUM TRAINING HEART RATE
220 – 33 (AGE) = 187
187 ÷ 75 (RESTING HEART RATE) = 112
112 × 0.50 (MINIMUM INTENSITY) + 75 (RESTING HEART RATE) = 131 BEATS/MINUTE